Healthy Habits for Life

BLAST YOUR BELLY FAT - 21 Powerful Habits to Lose Weight (Mini Habits, Increase Metabolism, Sleep Sound, Prevent Diabetes)

By Cathy Wilson

Copyright © 2015

Income Disclaimer

This book contains business strategies, marketing methods and other business advice that, regardless of my own results and experience, may not produce the same results (or any results) for you. I make absolutely no guarantee, expressed or implied, that by following the advice below you will make any money or improve current profits, as there are several factors and variables that come into play regarding any given business.

Primarily, results will depend on the nature of the product or business model, the conditions of the marketplace, the experience of the individual, and situations and elements that are beyond your control.

As with any business endeavor, you assume all risk related to investment and money based on your own discretion and at your own potential expense.

Liability Disclaimer

By reading this book, you assume all risks associated with using the advice given below, with a full understanding that you, solely, are responsible for anything that may occur as a result of putting this information into action in any way, and regardless of your interpretation of the advice.

You further agree that our company cannot be held responsible in any way for the success or failure of your business as a result of the information presented in this book. It is your responsibility to conduct your own due diligence regarding the safe and successful operation of your business if you intend to apply any of our information in any way to your business operations.

Terms of Use

You are given a non-transferable, "personal use" license to this book. You cannot distribute it or share it with other individuals.

Also, there are no resale rights or private label rights granted when purchasing this book. In other words, it's for your own personal use only.

Healthy Habits for Life

BLAST YOUR BELLY FAT - 21 Powerful Habits to Lose Weight (Mini Habits, Increase Metabolism, Sleep Sound, Prevent Diabetes)

By Cathy Wilson

Table of Contents

Introduction 9

17 Day Diet Basics 11

Powerful Benefits of Weight Loss 15

Phase 1 - Accelerate (Day 1-17)............................19

Phase 2 - Activate (Day 18-34) 25

Phase 3 - Achieve (Day 35-51) 31

Phase 4 - Arrive (Day 52+)....................................37

Strategies to Keep Fat off - Maintenance 41

Neat Food Factoids 49

The "Mental" of Dieting.......................................51

Physical and Dieting 55

Final Words 59

Bonus Chapter: 21 Powerful Habits to Lose Weight, Build Lean Muscle & Burn Belly Fat QUICKLY!.........61

Introduction

If you want to sum this diet up it's all about **LOSING WEIGHT FAST, BUILDING LEAN MUSCLE** and **MELTING BELLY FAT** for good!
Is this eating strategy perfect? Nope.
Am I perfect? Not even close.

Is this book going to help you blast fat fast and improve your health immensely? **YES! YES! YES!**
It's all about perspective. **YOU** choose the bits and pieces from all the information you ingest that are useful to improve your health.

Specifically this book focuses on the **17 Day Diet PLUS BONUS!**
How does the **17 Day Diet** work?

Sensibly using your natural body mechanics as a platform to get strong and lose weight. This eating strategy pays attention to your tolerances and preferences, what you enjoy and what you can't stand.

Of course these's always gonna be some "MUST DO" items if you're serious about blasting fat and turning on your sexy...

* Make healthier food choices
* Eat less calories than your body expends
* Fit physical activity into things you enjoy doing

As with each and every diet strategy out there, factors are in place delivering you to your desired weight loss within a specific time frame. If you know when to expect weight loss before you begin, it's perceived as **SUCCESS**.

The **17 Day Diet** sets you up for **SUCCESS**. If you've got 17 days to commit to following this plan you **WILL** lose fat and get one step closer to a healthier and happier you.

BONUS CHAPTER! 21 Powerful Habits to Lose Weight, Build Lean Muscle & Burn Belly Fat QUICKLY! (after final words)

Time to open your mind and turn on your determination so we can get started!

17 Day Diet Basics

This scientific based diet is broken down into 4 x 17 day cycles, which makes it easier to digest. Cleaning your house one room at a time is manageable. Trying to clean it spic and span in one shot is depressing and freaking crazy! While reading through this well-balanced and logical diet, keep in mind perspective. Take the information that makes sense to you. Open your mind to absorb and learn new tactics and strategies to help improve your health, and always look at the big picture. It's not about being right or wrong here, but if you choose the 17 Day Diet WILL fit.

The four main cycles in this diet are:
ACCELERATE
ACTIVATE

ACHIEVE
ARRIVE
The idea behind this lifestyle change is a common-sense approach is to teach your body how to run optimally with a few key and repetitive steps. First, to get rid of all the toxins and harmful chemicals in your body built up over time. Science says your body is not made to process anything but ALL NATURAL foods, which means sweet and tasty processed foods with zero nutrition and mountains of fat have no place to go.

Your body can't deal with chemicals, preservatives and bad fats, particularly in the oceanic amounts we eat them. Sodas, burgers, fries, chips, chocolate bars, cakes and pastries poison your body which interferes with each and every internal system. Stealing energy, triggering sickness and disease and making your life very depressing, often ending it pre-maturely.

Purging your system of this reservoir of poison makes sense.

Slowly with this practical eating style you add healthy and nutritious foods back into your system. Trying to show your body it can trust you and you do want to feed it premium fuel. The benefits are crazy fast weight loss, energy levels shooting up, minor ailments start to dissipate, chronic conditions take a turn for the better and preventative measures are in place to stay far away from serious disease. You also benefit your mental by looking and feeling better, which makes all the difference in the world. Measures are put into place to set you up for maintaining your weight loss and smart and energetic eating patterns, which is important if you really do are about you.

With this diet regular physical exercise is essential to make your results stick. It's not about exercising strenuously by any means, rather implementing daily physical activity into your schedule to help boost your metabolism and make your body work more effectively for you. With regular exercise your internal systems and your mental will both run more smoothly.

This is NOT a cyclical fad diet full of broken promises and inevitably broken scales. In basic, the 17 Day Diet is a concept of losing fat fast, gaining energy and deterring disease that is sensible and effective, a lifestyle move that will stick you are will to work for it. Habits are hard to break but this one is just too important to ignore. You matter.

My Thoughts . . .
It doesn't matter how you look at it. If you don't truly "want" to lose weight and get healthy, then please don't waste your time. When you are ready the 17 Day Diet will be ready and waiting to propel you to your weight loss goals fast.

This diet is all about sensible eating, diversity, control and reward, and implementing exercise regularly in a manageable and positive light. Talk about a plan destined to succeed!

Powerful Benefits of Weight Loss

It's essentially a universal fact that everyone on the face of this earth would like to drop at least a few pounds. Even those stick-pin models without an ounce of body fat want to get thinner! It's crazy, but true.

For most of us losing weight is a good thing. It's not just about that "feel good" feeling you get when you have to do your belt a notch tighter, or go shopping for a new dress because your old one just doesn't hug your curves anymore. Your body was programmed with what I call a "weight meter." This meter is set at your "ideal" weight. Meaning the point in which your body feels it functions optimally.

Of course this is different for each of us.
What happens over time through external factors is, we muck the safety mechanism up. We deprive ourselves of calories and sleep. Then overload it with fats and junk food. Back and forth like a ping pong ball causes our

meter to reset at an unhealthy weight, which naturally makes it even harder for us to drop fat even when we want to. We cause the negative interference.

Lucky for us we CAN lower our weight and reset our internal weight meter at a healthier weight if we commit to sensibly losing the weight and keep it off for at least 6 months. This is how long it takes for your body to trust you enough to believe you are finally going to keep your weight where it should, healthy and true.

Truth is if I was your body I wouldn't trust you either - would you?

Here are a few more befits of dropping fat and keeping it off!
* **Lengthens Life** -Studies show people that suffer from an obesity-related disease such as diabetes, have an increased length of life by losing weight and improved quality too.

* **Found Money** - By cutting out chips, cakes and expensive fast foods to lose weight, you're going to find lots and lots of money. Even if you just at removed one small bag of chips, one chocolate bar and one can of soda per week, that would save you about $144 per year!

* **Better Sex** - Experts agree that losing weight makes you more confident in your appearance and more likely to "feel" sexy. For men, obesity lowers testosterone levels, decreasing sex drive. By losing fat, testosterone levels jump and that's all good between the sheets.

* **Bring Forth the Energizer Bunny!** - Losing weight will literally take the weight of the world off your shoulders. Fat weighs you down physically and mentally. With the 17 Day Diet you will lose weight, gaining energy and pos-

16

itive life perspective throughout the process. The more fat that you lose, the more positives you gain.

Other Benefits include . . .
* Decreased cholesterol levels
* Lower blood pressure
* Better mobility and agility
* Increased respiratory function
* Less annoying aches and pains
* Better sleep
* More alert
* Increased productivity
* Better work relations
* Improved memory and cognitive capacity
* Lower blood sugar levels
* Decreased risk of diabetes, cardiovascular, cancer and other serious illness
* Less risk for depression and anxiety
* Increase in optimism
* Less wear and tear on skeletal system
* Improvement in circulation and internal system function
* Improved self-confidence and positive life direction
* Able to handle stress better

According to experts over SIXTY PERCENT of Americans are overweight or obese. That number scares the living crap out of me. Weight is something people can control and don't you think it's about time we started taking action? So much devastation, struggling and destruction goes hand-in-hand with obesity. The 17 Day Diet is a logical and sustainable option to turn your world right side up! It's up to YOU to pry your brain open to it.

My Thoughts . . .
Life is what you make it. Are you a positive or pessimistic person? I have no use for negativity, because it's magnetic in nature and will pull you in and stomp on you in

the blink of an eye. By making the choice to commit to changing your life for the better, to lose fat and keep it off, while gaining all sorts of other vital life benefits, you will experience just how fantastic life is.

The 17 Day Diet will help you establish new positive life perspective and make every single life challenge that much better for you. If you like to smile and feel good about yourself and life, or at least want to try, the 17 Day Diet will get you there.

Phase 1 - Accelerate (Day 1-17)

This first phase has the cards stacked against you simply because it's different. People DO NOT like change and find comfort in habit. Understand you will need to change your way of eating and perspective in exercising if you expect results. Wrap your head around this and you are definitely moving in the right direction.

The concept here is to lower your daily caloric intake down to around 1200 calories per day, shocking your system. Many people lose up to 15 pounds in this phase because of the change to your system. You are under-feeding your body, still within the healthy range, while gaining the trust and support of your body by fueling your system only with the essential vitamins and minerals it requires to function optimally. It's not going to be stressed anymore trying to purge your system of all the excess fats and toxins it's used to.

Did you know? There is such a thing as eating too little. If you don't give your body enough energy to at least match the energy demands you place on it, you

19

will force your body to shut down. What happens is your internal systems will flip into "starvation mode," because that's exactly what you are doing. This means any morsel of food you do eat is going to be stored as fat because your body doesn't trust you.

Your body doesn't know when you are going to feed it again so it is going to instinctively lower your metabolism, burn less calories and try to use as little energy as possible for your body function. For bonus points you're going to feel like crap too. By not fueling your body adequately you are forcing it to fight you in losing weight.

What is the bottom line? You've GOT to eat to lose weight!

With the 17 Day Diet you are restricting calories in this phase, but you aren't going so low that your body fights you with the weight loss battle. You are also cleverly setting yourself up for reward with this phase.

Understanding your psychosomatic or how your perceive things as just as important as the actions you're taking. How you think and feel is incredibly vital.

This diet phase has a built-in motivator to keep you going, a few to be more precise. The first is that you are going to see fast weight loss results and that will make you want more. Also you KNOW that in a few days you will be rewarded with more fuel for your body. You will be encouraged to eat more and this in itself is extremely motivational. Who doesn't want to eat more? The difference will be what you eat, when and how much. It's important you stay strong here because the last thing you want is to get lazy, feel defeated and fall back into the deadly trap of you "olden day" eating patterns.

Cycle 1 hydrates, cleanses, removes toxins and unhealthy carb traces from your physical system, while triggering the burning of fat and encourages a memory loss when it comes to unhealthy eating.

Exercising is critical with any long-term weight loss program. The 17 Day Diet plan sets you up for at least 17 minutes a day during both this first cycle and the next one. This exercising is very mild and can consist or just walking if you like. In the later cycles this strategy will shift gears.

Sample Foods Cycle One

The last thing we want to do here is make this lifestyle change confusing or difficult. Essentially you're encouraged to each lots of lean protein including chicken, beef, eggs and fish. Add to that, lots of healthy fibrous and nutritionally dense vegetables to start.

Low-fat no sugar and next to zero starchy carbs like white pasta, white bread and white rice is important. With cycle 1 you should consume a minimum of 2 probiotics each day with fresh fruits lowest in sugar, plums, berries and apples are examples.

Carbohydrate intake throughout this cycle comes from low sugar fruits and needs to be munched before two o'clock each day. For hydration and a boost to cleaning out your systems you should drink at least 8 ounces of warm lemon water upon waking, jumpstarting your digestive tract. Enjoying green tea at every meal is going to boost your metabolic process, while drinking 8 ounces of crystal clear water each day is going to make certain your fluids are running clear and your energy is optimal.

Vegetables to Cleanse
Asparagus, artichoke
Bell peppers, Brussels sprouts, broccoli
Celery, cauliflower, cabbage, carrots, cauliflower
Green beans and leafy green vegetables, garlic
Leeks, lettuce, kale
Onions, mushrooms and parsley
Spinach, scallions, tomatoes and watercress

Fruit- Fibrous - 2 portions each day
All berries, apples, oranges, grapefruit
Pears, plums, peaches, nectarines, red grapes

Lean Proteins
Chicken, skinless
Salmon, canned, broiled, grilled, baked
Tuna fish, water version
Lean turkey, skinless
Eggs, 2 per serving or 4 egg whites
Sole, catfish, flounder, fresh lake perch or bass

Probiotics - 2 portions each day
Sugar-free yogurt - 1 portion
Sauerkraut - 1/2 cup per serving
Acidophilous milk - 1 cup per serving
Kefir - 1 cup per serving
Yakult - 1 cup per serving
Fats 1-2 tbsp each day
Flaxseed or olive oil
Condiments – sparingly

Salsa, ketchup, sugar-free jams and jellies, low-fat sour
cream, fat-free salad dressing, salt, pepper, mustard,
spices, herbs, fat-free cheese, cooking spray, lite soy
sauce
Vegan Adjustments
1/2 cup tofu

2 vegetarian black bean burgers
1/2 cup beans or lentils
2 veggie sausage links
Up to 4 oz vegan cheese
2 scoops vegan rice protein powder
DAIRY SUBSTITUTIONS - 1 portion is one cup non-sweet soy, almond or rice milk. For yogurt use soy version

Sample Meals - 1200 calories per day
Day One
Breakfast
Hot lemon water
1/2 sugar-free yogurt
1 cup fresh berries
Green tea
Water

Lunch
Grilled chicken breast with two cups Romaine lettuce with tomatoes, carrots, celery and drizzle of low-fat salad dressing
Pear or apple sliced
Green tea
Water

Dinner
1 serving grilled salmon (4-6oz)
2 cups steamed veggies (asparagus, red, yellow and orange peppers)
Green Tea
Water

Snacks
1 cup carrots/celery
1/2 cup sugar-free yogurt

Day Two
Breakfast
Warm lemon water
2 boiled eggs
1 cup fresh fruit - oranges, grapefruit, red grapes
Green Tea
Water

Lunch
Grilled lean turkey breast
Mixed vegetables - broccoli, eggplant, artichoke
1 serving low-fat yogurt
Apple sliced
Green Tea
Water

Dinner
Can of tuna in water
2 cups spinach, carrots, radishes, celery, cucumber, drizzle low-fat salad dressing
Green Tea
Water

Snacks
1 cup mixed veggies
1/2 low-fat yogurt with 1/4 fresh berries
The idea here is to ensure you mix and match these healthy foods as you see fit. Gear it towards your preferences and tolerances and stick with the plan. During this first cycle you need to make huge adjustments in your eating. Lowering your daily caloric intake to 1200, boosting your fluid intake tremendously, and making sure you stick to the foods on the list, at least to start. Keep this first cycle eating and exercising for at least 17 minutes each day up and you will be all cleansed, energized and ready for cycle 2!

Phase 2 - Activate (Day 18-34)

In this phase you are re-activating your system, or rather starting it back up on a fresh new path. The food plan integrates a few more calories than Cycle 1. Think of it as your system being rewarded positively. Here you are keeping your metabolic process on its toes, thinking and guessing as to what you're going to throw at it next. This thought process maximizes the energy utilized which gets you fat loss results fast.

This switch in gears also helps to starve off boredom which just may be the number one cause of diet failure today. Although more than the previous phase the calorie intake is still low enough to continue on the path of weight loss, losing another 5-8 pounds on average with Phase 2. It's better than a sharp stick in the eye.

During this phase you're going to need to add 2 servings of natural starches every other day, eaten before 2 pm. Phase 2 lasts from day 18 to 34. Making sure you continue to focus on maximize your nutrients and minimizing calories with healthy, lean food choices that give your body the nutrients critical to optimal function. A learning process always and don't forget if you fall off the horse, recognize what you're doing and get your butt back up there pronto - no worries.

Sample Foods Cycle 2
Lean Protein
Shellfish (clams, oysters, mussels, scallops, shrimp)
Lean cuts beef (steak, ground beef)
Pork tenderloin, loin roast
Lamb sirloin roast, shanks
Veal

Starches - Complex Carbohydrates - Natural
Grains - 1 portion = 1/2 cup
Brown rice, bulgur, couscous, barley
Cream of wheat, grits, rice (long grain)
Quinoa, oatmeal
Black beans, kidney beans, lima beans, lentils
Soy beans, split peas, navy beans

Starches Vegetables
Potato - 1 portion = 1 medium
Sweet potato
Corn - 1/2 cup
Squash - 1 cup
Breadfruit - 1 cup

Cleansing Vegetables - same as Cycle 1
Fruits - Low- Sugar - same as Cycle 1
Condiments - same as Cycle 1

Fats - same as Cycle 1
Probiotics - same as Cycle 1

Sample Meals 1400-1500 Cal
Day One
Breakfast
Warm lemon water
1/2 cup sugar-free yogurt
1 cup fresh berries
1/2 cup grits with sweetener
Green Tea
Water

Lunch
Grilled pork tenderloin (4 oz)
2 cups mixed greens, tomatoes, carrots, radishes, corn, drizzle low-fat salad dressing
1/2 cup kidney beans
1 mango sliced
Green Tea
Water

Dinner
Sirloin steak (4 oz)
2 cup mixed veggies (broccoli, squash, 2 boiled eggs, eggplant)
Green Tea
Water

Snacks
1/2 cup quinoa
1 cup fresh fruit with 1/2 cup yogurt

Day Two
Breakfast
Warm lemon water
1/2 cup cream of wheat with 2 tbsp wheat germ

1/2 cup raspberries
1 pear sliced
Green Tea
Water

Lunch
1/2 cup sugar-free yogurt
1 cup blueberries
2 cups spinach, carrots, celery, onion, sprouts, tomato, drizzle fat-free salad dressing
1 boiled egg
Green Tea
Water

Dinner
4 large shrimp
1/2 cup brown rice
2 cups streamed vegetables (carrots, peas, broccoli, beans, peppers, water chestnuts)
Green Tea
Water

Snack
1/2 cup couscous with 1/2 cup peas/corn
1/2 cup yogurt with a peach

You should be feeling pretty good and getting used to watching what you eat and how much. The weight should continue to come off during this activation phase. It's important not to overdo it on the starches. There's more lenience with the lean protein and veggies, no cap except that you stay within the calorie range. Make sure you also continue with your 17 minutes per day of exercise. It doesn't have to be intense, but you do need to be consistent. If you are walking for your exercise make sure you walk 17 minutes EVERY DAY. If you are hiking or

biking, do the same. This is important for your health, re-sults and it's a part of a balanced lifestyle.
After 17 days in this Active phase or cycle you'll have graduated to Phase 3.

Phase 3 - Achieve (Day 35-51)

With the Achieve phase of this diet, you are looking to learn healthy eating habits which include portion control, regular eating times and always making healthy food choices that include foods dense in nutrients and not calories.

This phase allots you to have new foods to keep your body and mind guessing, increases the physical up to an hour each day and still limits your carbs to be in your tummy before 2 each day.

This cycle increases your overall caloric intake and decreases protein. Cutting protein consumption by at least a third is ideal. Now don't get too excited here, but now you can enjoy ONE alcoholic beverage per day, a 5 oz class of wine, bottle of beer or the standard 1.5 oz hard liquor drink. The two full servings of natural starches per day sticks can be eaten before 2 pm to make sure you don't start to plateau in weight loss.

You will keep with the same hydration process of warm lemon water in the morning, Green Tea each meal and plenty of cool refreshing water.
Calories should be around 1800.

Now is the time to get a touch more serious about exercise. Making sure you get in at least 40-60 minutes of intense aerobic exercise 3-5 times a week. This is a bit of an adjustment so you need to prepare yourself mentally and persevere. After a few weeks you will start feeling more comfortable and when combined with the positive results you're seeing, weight loss, energy gain, less aches and pains, improved self-confidence, you are going to get all fired up to work your body hard in these classes. Simply because you know the harder you work the faster you get results and it leaves you feeling fabulous!

Sample Foods Cycle 3
Lean Protein - same as Accelerate and Activate cycles.
Poultry to Add
Canadian bacon
Quail, pheasant, Cornish hen
Low-Fat lunch meat, bacon or sausage

Natural Starches
Whole grain breads
Pumpernickel and rye breads
Whole grain bagels and pitas (serving =1/2 portion)
Small whole grain tortilla

Cereals high in fiber (serving = 1 cup)
All-Bran
Cold cereals that are gluten-free
Granola that's low-fat, low-sugar (serving = 1/2 cup)
Fiber One
Vector

Pasta (serving = 1/2 cup)
Whole grain pasta
Vegetable pasta
High-fiber pasta
Pasta gluten-free

Vegetables - Unlimited
Cleansing veggies same as Accelerate and Activation cycles
Broccoli sprouts, alfalfa, cilantro, chilies, seaweed
Cactus, radishes, rhubarb, Swiss chard, yellow and green beans
Zucchini
Any other veggie you can think of

Fruits - 2 servings each day, 1 piece or 1 cup
All fruits from first 2 cycles
Cherries, bananas, apricots, figs
Papaya, kiwi, pineapple, tangerine
Any fruit

Probiotics
Same as first 2 cycles
Low-fat cheese - 1 serving = 2 ounces
Skim milk - 1 serving = 1 cup
Fat-free cottage cheese or ricotta cheese - 1 serving = 1/2 cup
Sugar-free almond, rice or soy milk for dairy-free - 1 serving = 1 cup

Fats - up to 2 tbsp per day
Avocado - 1/4 fruit
Canola or Walnut oil - 2 tbsp/serving
Light mayonnaise - 2 tbsp/serving
Nuts/seeds - 2 tbsp/serving
Low-fat margarine or dressing - 2 tbsp/serving
Full fat dressing or margarine - 1 tbsp/serving

Snacks under 100 calories
Low-fat Babybell cheese - 2 circles
Low-fat fruit bar or frozen yogurt
Low-fat granola bar
Plain microwave popcorn - 4 cups
Cheese string - 1 portion
Fat-free pudding - 1 cup

Sample Meals
Day One
Breakfast
Warm lemon water
One cup all bran cereal
One cup skim milk
1 cup fresh berries
Green Tea
Water

Lunch
1/2 cup low-fat cottage cheese
Banana
2 cups Romaine, carrots, celery, onions, 1/4 cup avocado, sprouts
1/2 cup couscous
Sliced Mango
Green Tea

Dinner
1 serving grilled sirloin steak
2 cups mixed steamed veggies (green/yellow beans, seaweed, peppers, zucchini)
1 cup low-fat yogurt
Green Tea
Water

Snacks
2 Babybell's

Whole grain granola bar

Day Two
Breakfast
Warm lemon water
4 egg whites
1 cup oatmeal
1 apple sliced
Green Tea

Lunch
Whole grain turkey sandwich (2 slices whole grain bread, 3-4 oz lean turkey, 2 tbsp light mayo, lettuce, tomato, cucumber, onion)
1 oz light cheese
Peach
Green Tea
Water

Dinner
Garden-Cheese salad (2 cups spinach, carrots, cucumber, radishes, carrots, tomato, 1/4 cup sunflower seeds, 1/4 cup fat-free cheese, drizzle fat-free salad dressing)
2 cups steamed veggies of your choice
1 cup vegetable soup
Green Tea
Water

Snacks
Small baked sweet potato
The achieve cycle is all about hitting the mark of what healthy eating and living is all about. By lowering your protein intake and increase calories you are deliberately switching gears to help keep your mind and body focused. The last thing you want to deal with when establishing new habits is a wandering mind.

By keeping starches and fruits before two, you are communicating to your body and internal systems that you want it to keep zapping fat calories so you can keep losing weight. Don't be shocked if your weight loss slows here because it should. Permanent weight loss has to cycle as the body would naturally and the 17 Day Diet plays it perfectly.

Adding up to an hour of intense cardio activity 3-5 days a week is going to ensure your body keeps losing weight. Expect about 5 pounds (give or take) during this cycle. Here you are getting used to the system. Don't expect perfect and allow for minor errors. This is the learning phase, fine-tuning will come later.

You should feel really good right now. Happy and proud of your progress and really getting used to all these positive life changes you have worked so hard to implement! Keep in mind it's always important for you to tailor each step to marry with your preferences and tolerances. If you are unsure of a specific food substitution or otherwise, make sure you ask an expert! Ask and you shall receive. Never give up, keep a healthy perspective and have patience, all key factors in your success! Up next is Phase 4!

Phase 4 - Arrive (Day 52+)

Consider yourself Arrived! Signifying that you have finally reached your destination, you've established personal-ized healthy eating habits and the focus here is learning how to make them stick. The last thing you want to do is regress backwards because you aren't thinking one step ahead of the game.

You feel fabulous right now, having lost the weight you wanted, energy levels are up, head is clearer and you are seeing a whole lot of sunshine in your world. With this phase you are going to keep shocking your system, mind and body, for continuous results. Stopping and starting your metabolism, giving it a little more than less, is going to ensure you don't plateau in the weight loss department or worse yet start sneaking the weight back on. This phase teaches you how to make sure that just doesn't happen.

By eating in a controlled but healthy fashion for five days and then allowing for a little bit "free-er" eating for two days, you're rewarding both your mind and body while forcing it to work efficiently and effectively for you.

So for the first 5 days make sure you eat meals that you would have in the first 3 cycles, controlled options. For the 6th and 7th day you will allow yourself a little bit extra, but no binging or out of control eating. An extra serving of fruit and veggies here or there, another snack or two, or perhaps an extra portion of whole grain toast with peanut butter is your treat. By now you will understand and appreciate how your body works and how rewarding "more" healthy eating can be.

You will actually get excited about having an extra up of fresh fruit with cottage cheese, or an extra serving of sweet potato fries on occasion. Having a beer or glass of wine with dinner is something you can work into your diet in moderation if that's something you really enjoy.

It's also important you still keep up your 60 minutes of intense cardiovascular exercise 3-5 days a week here to help strengthen and tone muscles, increase mobility, decrease aches and pains, burn fat, and give you that "feel good" shot of endorphins that will become addictive.
To ensure you have control here you should weight yourself on the weekend. If you see your weight isn't where it should be, immediately switch to one of your favorite cycles so you can get right back on track.

This isn't a one stop shop. The 17 Day Diet is a fabulous lifestyle that teaches you how to control your weight and reward yourself. A give-take relationship is all about learning and making adjustments where you see fit. There is no "right" or "wrong" here. It's about gaining

knowledge, reasonable perspective and expectations and perseverance. The only way you can fail with your new healthy 17 Day Diet lifestyle is to quit.
I'm telling you quitting is NOT an option because YOU ARE WORTH IT!

Strategies to Keep Fat off - Maintenance

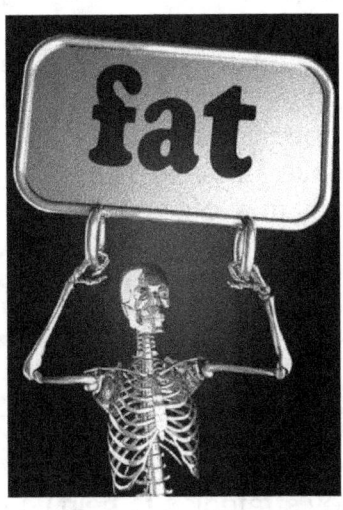

There aren't too many people that don't feel fabulous when they hit their weight loss goal. Agreed? Unfortunately we live in a society where Fad Diets are the norm, a billion dollar industry that fills people full of false hope and extreme strategies to drop fat fast. We want so badly to believe "magic fat blasting wands" really work, that we allow our emotion to override logic and actually believe that consuming only liquids for the rest of lives is a reasonable expectation. Obviously it isn't, and if we've lost 20 pounds fast drinking our nutrition, the second we start eating "real" food it all piles back on and we are depressingly back at ground zero. Don't tell me you can't relate here.

I really don't care what "eating strategy" you adopt to lose weight and get healthy. If it's extreme, lacks vital nutrients, doesn't take into consideration the natural rhythm of your body, regular physical exercise, and the ability to keep things interesting and diversified, you are eventually doing to derail and plummet over the edge.

* Reasonable expectations have to be set
* All nutrients must be included
* The terms and conditions or "rules" of your new eating strategy has to make sense to YOU
* You need to enjoy this routine of eating or learn to
* Your new eating strategy has to fit into your version of a healthy lifestyle, one you will learn to make habit and stick with for life

With The 17 Day Diet you and create the blueprint of positive nutrition that is going to better you mentally, physically and emotionally if that's what you choose. Here are a few key strategies to help you keep your excess weight off for good.

Support System
Why is it that we can so easily disappoint ourselves, often without a second thought? After so many failed weight loss attempts we seem to throw in the towel after our first misstep of "chowing" down a tub of triple chocolate ice cream when we're scheduled to be sweating up a storm at the gym, a cycle of disaster; extreme dieting and exercising, until we can't stand it anymore and surrender to a pig-out binge that depresses and devastates.

Having someone you trust to hold you accountable is a fantastic support to help keep you on track, particularly in the beginning where you are going to be challenged. This can be a friend or family member, maybe a nutritionist or eating group you've joined. Someone needs to be in place that will inspire you and won't listen to your whining. Rather they will positively fuel you to reach your weight loss goals and make sure you stay there. More than one support often works best.

Planning

By planning in everything you do a road is created that leads you to success. Planning is productive and increases the chances you're going to reach your goal. A house can't be built without planning. A Christmas dinner isn't going to run smoothly without a master plan of attack.

The same goes with the 17 Day Diet. If you don't plan out and know what you're going to eat and when BEFORE it's time to eat, there's going to be trouble. This could leave you starving and more willing to snack when you're trying to figure out what to make. Worse yet you may grab something you shouldn't be eating just because you can't be bothered to run to the grocery store to get food. I think you see where I'm headed here.

Plan your meals at least 2-3 days in a row so that when your tummy tells it's time to eat you don't have to use your brain cells to figure out what. If you are really organized and can buy all your groceries on Sunday for the week, that's even better.

Measuring Routinely

As humans we need to see and measure progress as incentive to keep on going. If you are a runner, you will time yourself to see if get faster with the adjustments you've made in your training. The time is a measuring tool.

When it comes to losing weight and getting healthy there are lots of tools people use to measure. Some just go by how their clothes fit. If they're starting to get snug action needs to be taken. Others may tune into their body and go by how they are feeling.

The most accurate and level way to keep on track with your hard-earned weight loss is to step on the scale periodically. This is the quickest route to making sure you're maintaining your weight and lifestyle changes.

Notice - Weighing yourself too often isn't a good thing because your body needs time to shed fat and work through the cycle. Weighing yourself once a week on the weekend is plenty. Trying weighing yourself with the same clothes on at the same time, so that you get a little more accurate reading. In your birthday suit really is the best, but I'll leave that one up to you.

Taking body fat measurements also works. Just make sure you are using the tape measure accurately and this method is best with the scale too. Once every two weeks is plenty.

Journals also work great where you record your days in detail. Examples would be: How you were feeling, what you ate, the pounds lost and so forth. This gives you something concrete to look back on whenever you like to remind you of just how far you've come, how much progress you've made.

By making a habit of recording your progress and even your setbacks, you're much more likely to hold yourself accountable to you.

Use Your Crystal Ball

It's important to troubleshoot where you can. Perhaps you have some people you hang out with that choose to eat unhealthy and won't take no for an answer. Maybe you need to steer clear of them while you're getting yourself established with the 17 Day Diet?

You may be programmed to always have snacks at the Saturday afternoon show. Improvise by making sure you eat before you go. Maybe you can work in 4 cups of your own popcorn for a snack and can treat yourself to a diet Green Tea, opting for some sugar-less gum instead of chips and candy during the show. Theater popcorn is very bad for you, so just don't make it an option. Where there's a will there's a way and if you use your crystal ball you're going to be successful.

Accept You're Human
So what? You had a couple squares at the party or ended up having a serving of mashed potatoes at 6pm. Let it go. You're human and life happens. The important factor here is that you realize what you did and just need to tighten up the strings a little and get right back on track. You will find the further along you get on the 17 Day Diet the more forgiving your body will be.

A great method of counteracting any damage done with an eating mistake is to throw in some extra exercise. Remembering this is all about give and take. So you had 3 light beers at a friend's party when you should have had just one? No worries! That's about 200 extra calories, by adding 30 minutes extra of moderate biking you will level the playing field. This sort of thinking is invaluable when looking to maintain your gains.

This strategy can be executed by cutting back a little on each of yours meals after you've had a few too many calories. Remembering it you back your calories too much this will force your body to battle you in fat loss.

Increase Activity Outside of Eating

Remember, out of sight, out of mind. By keeping yourself busy with hobbies and other interests, you're not going to me so focused on good. If you don't have any hobbies get some. Think of things you've always wanted to try and get to them. Maybe you want to learn how to paint, roller-skate, bowl or play bingo. The idea here is to get more involved and interested in all the life has to offer to fill the food void you may have been focused on at one time. Change is good.

Diversify

This is the spice of life. Diversity keeps things exciting and when it comes to maintaining weight loss, diversity is king! Mixing up the foods you are eating and the exercise you are doing is going to push your body to burn more calories and keep yourself from slipping into boredom because you're going to always have to be sharp in thinking.

If you catch yourself getting a little too much into routine, that's your cue to make a few minor adjustments, which can be as simple as picking up the pace in your walk for five minutes and then back down to normal for the remainder.

Reward Yourself

We work for reward in everything and if it's missing, veering off course is more likely to be a reality. If you lose 15 pounds after Phase 1 you should reward yourself for your efforts. Treat yourself to a new pair of pants, a specialty Green Tea at the new coffee shop, or maybe you're a "shoe-a-holic" and with each goal a new pair of shoes goes into your closet.

It doesn't matter how big or small your reward, just make sure you do recognize and reward your efforts regularly.

That's incentive to move forward full speed ahead.

My Thinking . . .
Having a maintenance plan in place is critical with the 17 Day Diet and any other newly established eating strategy for that matter. Why would you want to risk gaining all your fat back and falling back into your old and unhealthy eating? Prevention is the key and having a maintenance plan in place will remind you of all the positive health changes you are making.

Your health and wellness is too important to ignore and maintenance is a must for long-term success.

Neat Food Factoids

Food is something we all have in common. Here are some weird and interesting food facts that may be news to you.

- Peanuts are technically legumes and not nuts. They're also used to make dynamite!
- It may not surprise you that Coke was originally green.
- Ketchup was sold in the early 1800s as medicine.
- Coconut water can be used as blood plasma in emergencies because it's sterile and has a compatible PH.
- The first recorded soup was hippopotamus.
- Vinegar has the ability to melt pearls.
- Carrots were initially grown for "Karoto" medicine by the ancient Greeks.
- Worcestershire sauce is made from anchovies dissolved in vinegar.
- Avocados are poisonous to birds and contain the most protein of any fruit.
- Spam will last for eternity in an unopened can.
- Grapes explode in the microwave. It's true!

- Cherries are a part of the rose family.
- Bananas technically aren't a fruit, they're an herb.
- If you bounce a cranberry high it's ripe to eat.
- Ears of corn will always have an even number of rows.
- The darker the pumpkin shell the longer it lasts

My Thoughts . . .
This was just a few neat food facts to add to your
knowledge base. Information is knowledge and
knowledge is power, useful or otherwise.

The "Mental" of Dieting

Having a positive mental attitude in anything is important. When it comes to dieting and the 17 Day Diet, a positive attitude will set you up for success. Positive thinking is what carries you through those "tough" days where you just can't seem to muster up the energy you'd like. Those times where you happen to be feeling down or blue, things just aren't going as planned, this is where conscious positive mental thinking will make the world of difference.

It's learned and takes time, patience and commitment. Anyone can start a diet plan and be all excited initially. This wears off fast and having positive thinking is only going to help you stick with it faithfully for the long haul. I daresay the most important component of a diet plan is a positive mindset.

Your Mental and the 17 Day Diet Plan
The mind is a powerful thing and if you think it you can do it. Your thoughts are what dictate your actions and often

just putting random things into your head are the beginnings of a new reality to be. Think of the "thought" as the seed in the garden. Without the seed, you will never have a beautiful flower. Without committing to the healthy eating strategies of the 17 Day Diet with a positive mental attitude, you'll have a tough time sticking with it for good. Positive thinking means you aren't going to quit and you'll be able to overcome any barriers that pop up, particularly the emotional and truly powerful ones.

Positive Mental Thinking will Keep you on Track

If you program your head to be positive you are always going to keep things around you to keep you focused and determined to reach your weight loss goals. Maybe there's a cute little black dress you really want to fit into. Your positive mental thinking will remind you that is the first thing you're going to purchase WHEN you drop the weight.

Maybe you are running for your cardio exercise in Phase 3 and really find the last 15 minutes challenging. Your positive thinking will override this negativity and remind you there's a huge ice cold bottle of lemon water waiting for you when you finish.

A positive head is a focused head, one that will create an environment where you are inevitably going to succeed.

Helps Relate Positive to Dieting

We are conditioned to associate "dieting" with negative. Deprivation, no energy, starvation, and all sorts of other depressing thoughts naturally pop up when you hear the word diet.

This is all in our head, it's a matter of perception and if you consciously choose to see the good in things you will.

Your reality is what you make it. If you tell your mind that dieting is not a negative thing and that it's all about making positive changes that will better you and your life, you WILL believe it and it WILL happen. All you've got to do is focus on it and believe.

Ensures you Surpass Emotional Hurdles
Emotional eating is the causal factor for many overweight people. Many don't even realize they are eating when they aren't even hungry. They've created a habit to grab chips when they are depressed after getting dumped. Or if they have a bad day at work an ice cream on the way home is short-term therapy. Sure it may boost your spirits short term with a fast injection of sugar into your system. Sadly it's short-lived and you have a depressed feeling and the guilt of unhealthy eating to deal with.

Studies show happier people are less depressed and have a decreased likelihood of eating because of their emotions, or in the least, learning how to recognize the triggers and control them. The key here for losing weight and sticking to your 17 Day Diet weight loss strategy.

My Thoughts . . .
When you are thinking in a positive light you are focused on sunshine. Success is something you strive towards rather than make excuses to never get there. With a little time and patience and whole lot of persistence you will make positive thinking a staple for you and this is going to push you though to the finish line of each and every one of your weight loss and life goals.

Physical and Dieting

Your body was built to be physical EVERY DAY. It's pro-grammed into your genes and when you deny your body by lazing on the couch and driving when you could be walking, you are only harming your health.

Each of your internal systems that control your emotional, physical and mental are reliant on an intricately timed group of systems. These systems run more efficiently and effectively with regular exercise. "You snooze- you lose" when it comes to moving your body. If you choose not to exercise you'll lose mobility and agility, clear think-ing and energy, aches and pains will become your focus and routine daily activities will require pain and huge ef-fort.

Establishing healthy and sensible eating with the 17 Day Diet, combined with regular physical exercise is exactly what will set you up for permanent weight loss and a long and healthy life.

Other exercise benefits are:

* *Decrease Risk of Serious Disease* - Exercising regularly as the 17 Day Diet encourages will help lower your chances of developing serious disease. Heart disease, stroke, diabetes and various cancers are a few common ailments exercise can deter.

* *Lowers Blood Pressure* - A risk factor of cardiovascular disease and stroke is high blood pressure. Regular exercise lowers blood pressure and cholesterol naturally.

* *Reduction of Aches and Pains* - Many of us just assume aches and pains are "normal." By taking care of your body with regular physical exercise you will immediately notice many of your "usual "aches and pains will magically disappear.

* *Lower Back Pain* - Routine physical exercise will naturally strengthen back muscles, improve circulation, release "feel good" hormones and help to alleviate lower back pain without harmful medications. If you can provide pain relieve naturally and prevent progression, why wouldn't you?

* *Endorphin Release* - Exercise that gets your heart rate up naturally releases endorphins (hormones) which boost your spirits long after you've finished exercising. These chemicals help to mask pain and leave you feeling energetic and positive. Many, including me, believe these chemicals are addictive, and it's all good.

* *Triggers Metabolic Boost* - Of course a highlight of exercise is boosting the calories burned and this means if you are eating the right foods, fat loss will be increased. Regular physical exercise with smart eating like the 17 Day Diet is going to speed up the rate in which you lose

fat AND boost your positive perspective, a double win for you.

Improves Mobility - Routine physical exercise naturally improves motility and leaves you mobile longer. If you are moving around more you will be "able" to do this longer. If you are stuck in a chair day after day without exercise, eventually you will lose the ability to walk or move without pain. It's your choice to get moving or else!

My Thoughts . . .
The 17 Day Diet includes regular physical activity from the start. It's important to start slow and work your way up, listen to your body and always check with your doctor before beginning just to be safe.

Exercising regularly improves you mentally, physically, emotionally and socially, all positively. Keeping it diverse and exciting will starve off boredom and force your body to give you results fast, never hitting a plateau and always reaching your weight loss goals sooner not later. Ideally 45 minutes to an hour 3-5 days a week works. It's important for you to find what works for you and make it habit.

Final Words

As mentioned previous there is no "perfect" diet or exercise program. There's always room for improvement and you need to make the adjustments necessary in each to make them "fit" your tolerances and preferences.

What works for your best friend, may not work for you and that's okay. You owe it to yourself to use the 17 Day Diet and make it work for you. Tweak it where you need to and find your rhythm. This diet is the fastest route for you to lose fat, gain energy, increase motility and agility, deter disease, and make better of the symptoms you might be suffering from any chronic conditions.

The 17 Day Diet is going to teach you a sensible strategy to giving your body the right amount of vitamins and minerals to run optimally, while allowing you to control your weight loss. Fast and effective is what the 17 Day Diet is. All that's left now is for you to experience it.

Bonus Chapter: 21 Powerful Habits to Lose Weight, Build Lean Muscle & Burn Belly Fat QUICKLY!

Why should you want to burn belly fat?
According to fitness expert *Jennifer Cohen,* belly fat is the most dangers fat of all! All sorts of diseases are associated with a larger girth. And it takes a heck of a lot more than a few zillion crunches and other abdominal exercises to shrink your belly down.

Also keep in mind it's not just your poor food choices and lack of exercise that expand your waistline. STRESS is a HUGE contributing factor to storing fat around your waist. I'm going to help you BLAST belly for good with 21 Effective and Powerful habits to lose weight, build lean muscle & burn pesky belly fat FAST!

Habit 1 - INTERVAL TRAINING - *Men's Fitness* experts report the most effective route to build your body strong and lose weight is to interval train with strength training, weight training, and cardiovascular activity.

Interval training is all about keeping your mind and body guessing with different exercises, intensity levels, rep counts, duration and combinations. This forces your body to burn the maximum number of calories because "lazy" isn't in the picture.

The constant changes allow you to workout for shorter periods of time with maximum benefit. You work hard and get results fast.

Great examples of intense fat blasting interval training are cross-training, bootcamp group sessions, and circuits.

30-35 minutes 4-5 days a week should do the trick!

Habit 2 - BREAK UP EXERCISE - Research shows there's an advantage to breaking your workout up throughout the day. This works great when you've got a busy schedule. By exercising 10 minutes in the morning, afternoon, and early evening, you are encouraging your body to keep your fat blasting metabolism up all day, and not just during and shortly after exercising.

It really doesn't matter how you get it. Just make sure you get your 30-45 minutes of intense exercise in one way or another daily.

Habit 3 - SLEEP - Make sure you shut your body down every night routinely and get the quality 7-8 hours your body needs to function optimally. If you are skimping out on sleep you're mucking up your biorhythm. This triggers cortisol levels to skyrocket, sugar cravings to increase, insulin sensitivity to kick in, and belly fat to start growing! Chemical is chemical. Get the sleep your body needs each night and lose weight in the process.

Habit 4 - DON'T STARVE YOURSELF - Extreme tactic aren't going to work here. If you aren't providing your body with the minimum number of calories it requires to function daily, it WILL fight you.

*You'll have no energy
*Your body will burn muscle instead of fat
*Your metabolism will slow
*Your body will try and store every calorie you do eat as fat
*Your body will restrict calories used
When your body isn't getting enough calories it drops into starvation mode. Making it extra hard to lose weight. You've got to eat to lose weight!

Habit 5 - PUMP IRON - *Women's Day* fitness experts say building lean muscle by strength training and weight lifting goes a long in shrinking your size, toning up, and losing weight. Muscle building also increases your resting metabolism. So you burn more calories even when napping if you've got lean muscle!

Habit 6 - PROTEIN/CARB COMBINATION - *Mayo Clinic* specialists report eating servings of lean protein and complex carbs before and after exercising provides the energy to burn fat and build muscle, and supports recovery.

The protein provides the energy for muscle building and the carbs give you the long term energy to workout longer.
*Apple with peanut butter
*Egg with whole grain toast
*Yogurt with fresh fruit
*Half a peanut butter sandwich on whole grain bread
*Handful of nuts and banana
*Small garden salad with chicken breast
Those are a few great snacks before and after working out!

Habit 7 - EAT ENOUGH PROTEIN - Nutrition experts at *Fit Magazine* say if you don't provide your body with 2-3 servings of complete protein every day you may be protein deficient.

If your body doesn't have the protein available for energy it will use the muscle you have.

Protein isn't something your body makes and it can't be stored. This means you need to eat your protein every day if you want to blast belly fat, build muscle, and get lean and sexy!

Habit 8 - MEASURE YOURSELF - Dr. Carol Shively, Wake Forest School of Medicine, says you need to lose belly fat if you're a woman with a waist measurement of more than 35 inches, 40 inches for men.

Make a habit of pulling out the measuring tape monthly to keep on track!

Habit 9 - LOSE WEIGHT EVERYWHERE - *WebMD* reminds us we really can't target fat loss. In order to lose belly fat you've got lose it all over. Now you can "tone" your belly area but that's not losing belly fat. So don't be fooled.

Habit 10 - ELIMINATE PROCESSED FOOD - By getting rid of high fat low nutrient processed food you are cutting a huge number of fat and calories from your diet. Often it's best to ease into this habit because an all-or-nothing approach may backfire.

If you usually grab a burger, fry and shake for lunch, opt for a salad instead of the fry, or a milk instead of the milkshake. One step at a time and you WILL get there!

Habit 11 - UP YOUR FIBER - Studies at *WebMD* report people eating at least 10 grams of soluble fiber per day have less tummy fat over time than other people. Make sure you get at least 6-8 servings of fresh fruits and veggies per day and you should do just fine.

Habit 12 - DE-STRESS - Everyone's got stress. How you handle yours is important. **medicinenet.com** researchers say that stress may be partially responsible for weight gain because stress can cause your hormones to go out of whack, which triggers weight gain.

Great ways to remove stress are:
*Sex
*Exercise
*Meditation
*Vacation
*Enjoying nature
*Getting some sun exposure

Habit 13 - EAT HIGH CALORIE FOOD IN MODERATION - When you are going to indulge don't go crazy. Try eating a fresh bowl of berries with a dollop of real whipped cream, a sprinkle of cheese on your salad instead of drowning it, or a bite of chocolate cake instead of the whole thing.

This habits will take willpower and persistence. You CAN do it if you want to!

Habit 14 - DRINK WATER - Sugary fruit juices, soda, and energy drinks doesn't do anything for your waistline and certainly isn't helping you lower your risk of developing diabetes. By training yourself to drink more water, 6-8 glasses every day, you are hydrating your body to run optimally, reducing calories, and energizing yourself to blast fat.

A great habit to get into is carrying a water bottle with you throughout the day and making sure you fill it up at least twice!

Habit 15 - SMALLER PLATES - According to *Readers Digest* studies, downsizing your dinner plate will help you feel fuller and eat less. Do the same think with your drinks and you'll help reduce your total calories and blast belly fat!

The mind is a powerful thing!

Habit 16 - EAT RAW - Processing destroys essential nutrients and adds all sorts of harmful chemicals, toxins, and calories to your food. Choosing to eat raw when you can naturally eliminates calories so you can lose weight. Make sure you have raw food on your plate each meal because this will also up your fiber intake, helping you feel fuller longer.

Habit 17 - SERVE FOOD RESTAURANT STYLE - Studies show that by simply serving your meal on a plate, rather than on dishes and bowls on the table, you're less likely to go for seconds habitually.

Breaking a habit is tough but you've got to start somewhere. Learn to pay attention to what you're eating and ask yourself if you're still hungry, or just eating more because it's there.

Habit 18 - EAT AS MANY VEGGIES AS YOU LIKE - Making a habit of eating as many fresh veggies as you like is a good thing. There may be times where you meal hasn't quite filled you up. If that's the case, train yourself to first take another serving of more veggies.

Vegetables are loaded with protective antioxidants, fiber to help you feel full and regular, plenty of vitamins and minerals, and they are low in calories, essential in losing weight fast!

Habit 19 - NO MORE WHITE FOOD - White bread, pasta and rice are simple sugar foods that are loaded with sugar, very little fiber and even less nutrients. They provide energy that's short term and are directly linked with obesity, belly fat, and all sorts of serious disease.
Making a habit of avoiding white food is a smooth move to help you lose belly fat. Opt instead for complex carbohydrates. Whole grain breads, cereals and rice are chalk full of essential vitamins and minerals, fiber, and help you sustain energy longer.
Great complex carb food choices are...
*Legumes
*Whole grain bread, bagels and pitas
*Whole wheat pasta and rice
*Beans
*Other fresh veggies

Habit 20 - CHEW SLOWLY - According to experts at *WebMD*, by taking the time to consciously pay attention to each bite you take, you're much more likely to experience satisfaction with less. Of course that's only going to help you shrink your scales number and blast belly fat. Start with a "20 chew rule" for each bite. This forces you to take longer to eat, and increases the chance you're going to eat a heck of a lot less!

Habit 21 - START WITH BREAKFAST - Studies show people that make a healthy habit of starting their day with breakfast, have lower body weights overall, and less belly fat than people that skip the most important meal of the day.

You don't drive your car on empty and you shouldn't do the same to your body. In order to lose weight and belly fat you've got to eat. And by having a healthy breakfast with lean protein and complex carbs, you are setting your mind and body up for FAST weight loss!
Apply these healthy habits and start blasting your belly fat today!

Last Thoughts…

*THANK-YOU for reading my masterpiece. I hope you learned a little something, or at least got a few smiles.
*I would appreciate a millisecond or three of your time for a quick review, to help me build my masterful book empire higher.
*Whatever you do, don't forget to smile, and of course, check out my website for more of my e-Book masterpieces at: www.flawlesscreativewriting.com

Cathy ☺